Amazing Health Benefits of Intermittent Fasting

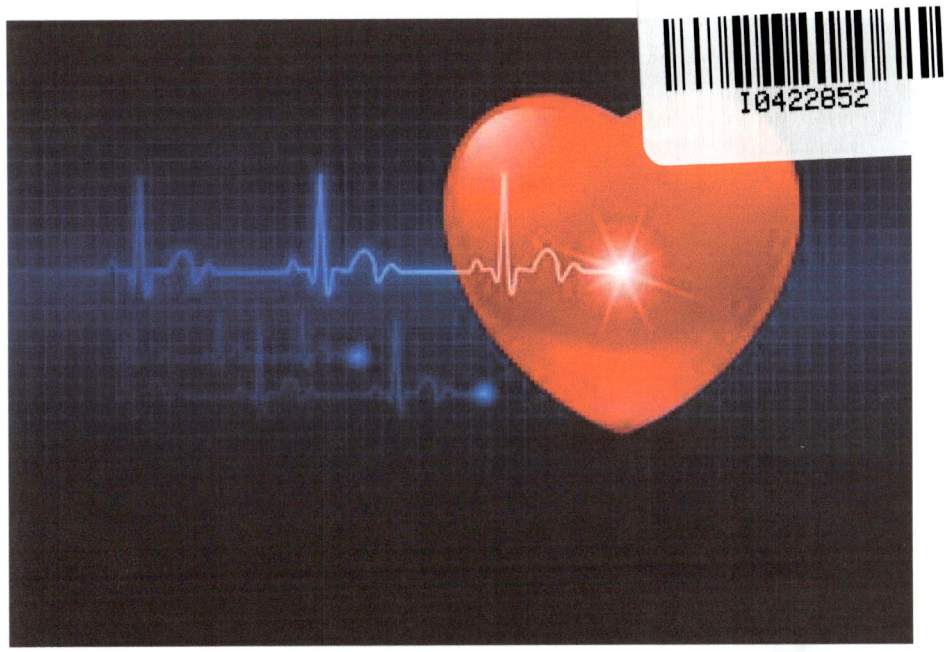

By M. Usman

Health Learning Series

Mendon Cottage Books

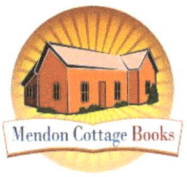

JD-Biz Publishing

Disclaimer

The information is this book is provided for informational purposes only. It is not intended to be used and medical advice or a substitute for proper medical treatment by a qualified health care provider. The information is believed to be accurate as presented based on research by the author.

The contents have not been evaluated by the U.S. Food and Drug Administration or any other Government or Health Organization and the contents in this book are not to be used to treat cure or prevent disease.

The author or publisher are not responsible for the use or safety of any diet, procedure or treatment mentioned in this book. The author or publisher is not responsible for errors or omissions that may exist.

Warning

The Book is for informational purposes only and before taking on any diet, treatment or medical procedure it is recommended to consult with your primary care provider.

Our books are available at

1. Amazon.com

2. Barnes and Noble

3. Itunes

4. Kobo

5. Smashwords

6. Google Play Books

Table of Contents

Preface

There are different dieting plans present in the world today which can be obtained through different resources. Each of these dieting plans claims to be better than the other one. But the plan mentioned in this book makes no such claims. It is about a popular plan or you should say a complete way of eating and living known as "Intermittent Fasting". Now you might be wondering what is intermittent fasting, what are its benefits and how to apply it in your own life? But wait a minute. Just take a deep breath. If the answer to all these queries would have been this easy, I would have just sufficed on writing an article and not a whole book on the topic. You will just have to read this book to get your queries answered.

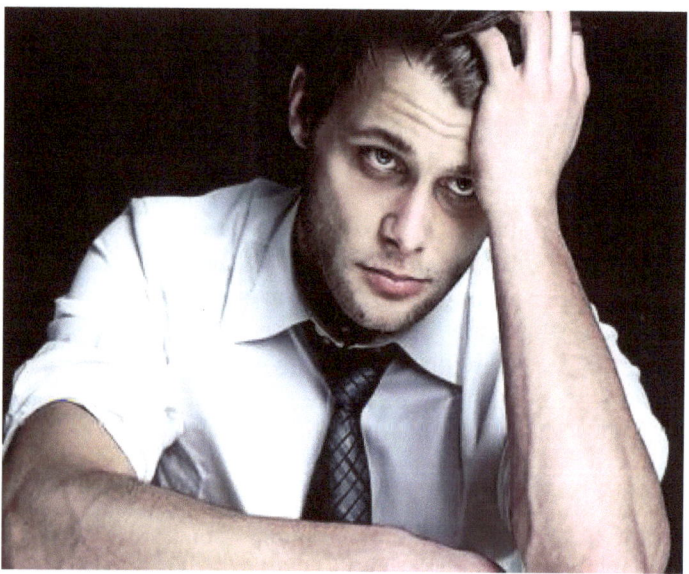

Before formally starting the topic, a brief overview of the book will give the readers a better idea about the book. As the title suggests, the focus of this book is to answer only one question and it is that what are the health benefits of intermittent fasting? However, other aspects are also discussed in the book. This book can be divided into three parts. The first part will give a brief introduction about intermittent fasting like what it is, the mechanism behind it and how to apply it in your everyday life? The second portion analyzes the pros and cons of intermittent fasting and ways to maximize its benefits. The third part will discuss the health benefits (the main focus of this book) of intermittent fasting.

So, as of this moment, the choice is yours. You can either throw it away just by reading the introduction because it doesn't fascinate you much or you can read through the whole book. But let me just say one thing. After reading this book, you will be happy that you came across something this good.

SECTION 1: INTERMITTENT FASTING: AN INTRODUCTION

CHAPTER 1: How It Works?

What Is Intermittent Fasting?

Intermittent fasting can be defined simply as an alternation between fasting (time when you aren't allowed to eat) and non-fasting periods (time when you are allowed to eat). The question of how long the fasting period is depends upon the type of fasting plan you have chosen. Each of the plans has its own specific benefits and normally the fasting period lasts from a minimum of 16 to 36 hours. An example will further clarify the concept of intermittent fasting. Suppose a person who is doing intermittent fasting might fast 16 hours and eat in the remaining 8 hours.

Mechanism and Working behind Intermittent Fasting:

Now that you have some understanding of intermittent fasting, you would better understand the mechanism behind it.

The main source of the body fuel is glucose which can be obtained from three energy sources namely carbohydrates, proteins and fats. The easiest way to obtain glucose is from carbs (carbohydrates) whereas the hardest way is from fats. So firstly all the energy is obtained from the carbohydrates; it is only after the glucose reserves run out that the body makes use of the fats, converting them into glucose and thus providing energy to the body.

Now that you have an understanding about the energy sources of the body, let us see what happens when we eat food. The calories produced after eating are first stored in the body in the form of glycogen. When the glycogen reserves are filled, the remaining calories are stored in the body in the form of fat. In normal circumstances, when a person eats six meals a day, the glycogen reserves never run out because of continuous supply of calories. And our body never gets a chance to burn its fat reserves.

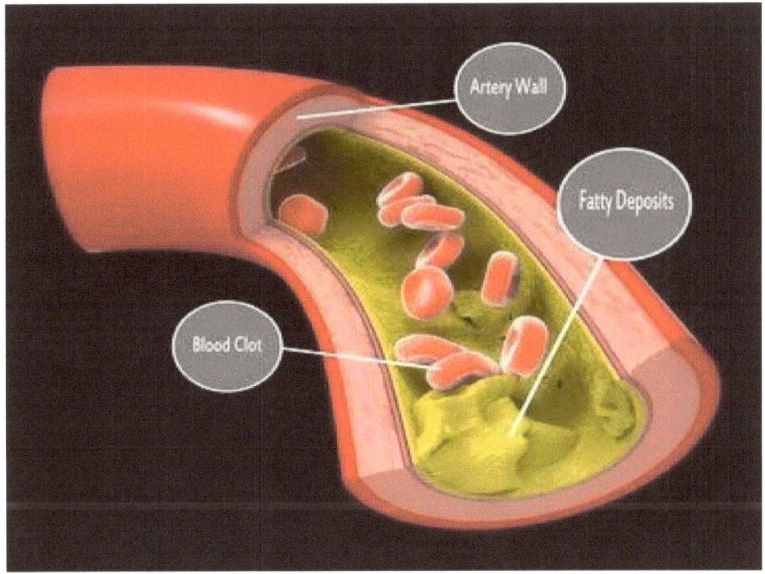

On the other hand what happens when a person doesn't eat food or in other words the person fasts? The body has to use the stored energy to keep the things going smoothly. First the glycogen reserves are called upon and glycogen is broken down to form glucose. When the reserves of glycogen deplete, it is only then that body starts to use other sources of energy like fats.

Now let us go at micro level to have a better understanding of intermittent fasting. After eating, glucose is released in the body which basically increases the blood sugar level in the body releasing a hormone known as "insulin", the main function of which is the removal of sugar from the blood and store it in the liver in the form of glycogen. First, all the extra glucose gets stored in the form of glycogen and if still enough glucose is left it is shunted to the fat synthesis pathway. Opposite happens during fasting, the levels of insulin fall and a hormone known as HSL (Hormone Sensitive Lipase) is released which is responsible for the conversion of fats to fatty acids and energy thereafter.

In a crux, during fasting, the glucose obtained from carbs run out quickly and the body uses the stored glycogen and fats for the synthesis of glucose. Fat burning can't happen when a person six meals a day because more and more calories are obtained from food. Instead of fats being used for energy, more and more fats start being stored in the body.

Chapter 2:

Does It Really Work Or Another Way To Rob Your Money?

So you might be wondering that does intermittent fasting really work or is it just another of many ways to rob you of your money. Now I can keep on boasting about how beneficial this diet plan is but it won't be that convincing. Some statistics and researches mentioned in the following paragraphs will be all it takes to get you interested in intermittent fasting.

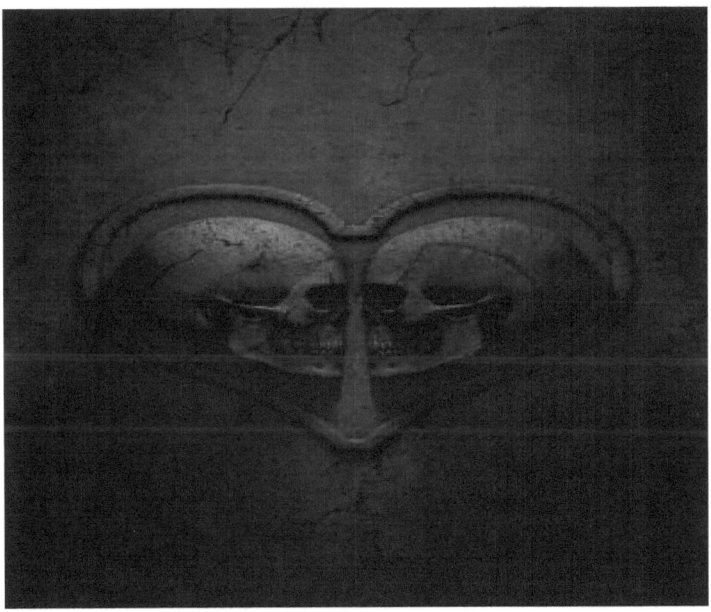

Before going into the details of these studies, one thing should be kept in mind by the reader. Intermittent fasting is economically beneficial. The reason behind this is simple. In this diet plan, a person fasts during the maximum time of the day and eats only for a few hours. So a person has to make the eating schedule for the eating hours only. On the other hand, in other diet plans a person has to make a schedule for 24 hours which increases the costs. So intermittent fasting is highly cost effective in comparison to other diet plans.

Studies Supporting Intermitting Fasting:

A recently reported research by biologist Satchidananda Panda and his colleagues at Salk's Regulatory laboratory has further clarified the situation. In the research, the laboratory team fed a high-fat and high-caloric diet to mice but altered the timings of their eating. The mice were divided into two groups one of which was given access to food 24 hours a day while the other group had access to food for only eight hours during the night time. The results showed that mice that ate only eight hours didn't develop problems like high blood pressure and chronic inflammation. On the other hand, mice who had access to food all day became more obese and developed different health problems like higher cholesterol, metabolic diseases and high blood sugar level.

Now let us move towards human studies. A clinical study published in 2007 showed significant alleviation of the symptoms of asthma and inflammation in 9 patients who followed the intermittent dieting plan. The patients fasted every other day for two weeks.

In another study, which was conducted by Mark Mattson, a senior investigator for the National Institute on Aging, it was shown through experimentation that overweight patients lost eight percent of their body weight when they cut their caloric intake by as much as 80% on alternate days.

The above mentioned studies prove the fact that intermittent fasting has various health benefits for humans.

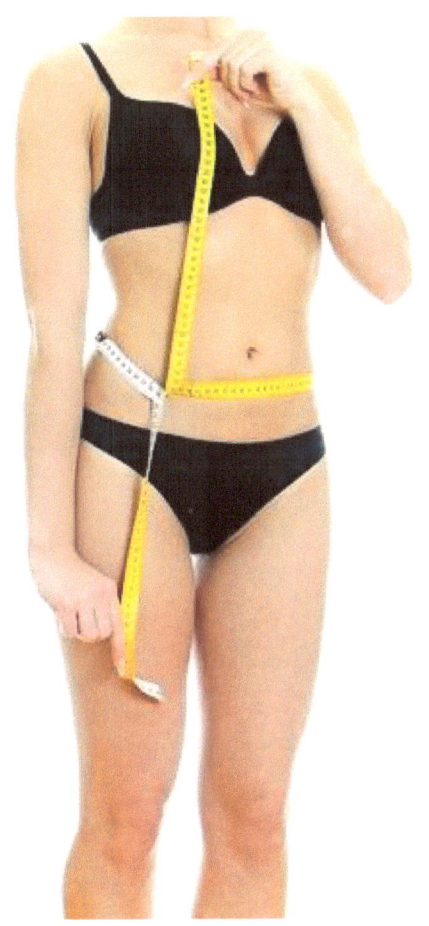

Conflicting Studies:

The above paragraphs have shown the researches in support of intermittent fasting. However, as with other dieting plans, conflicting studies are also present in intermittent fasting. A study published in 2011 on rats has shown that long term intermittent fasting leads to an increase in the blood sugar level. Moreover, another study published in 2010 showed that rats fasting regularly mysteriously developed stiff heart tissues which decreased the heart's ability to pump blood to the body.

In a crux, the conflicting studies on intermittent fasting are not as numerous as compared to those in support of intermittent fasting. A vast majority of dieticians and experts are in support of intermittent fasting dieting plan and you should also definitely give it a try. So what's the wait! Turn the pages over.

Section 2: Intermittent Fasting Specifics

Chapter 3: Pros of Intermittent Fasting

By now, you might have guessed that this dieting plan is very beneficial. This chapter will inform you about some pros of intermittent fasting.

The main benefits of this dieting plan are as follows:

- The first benefit of intermittent fasting is that it simplifies your life. You no longer have to cook and plan for 6 meals a day. You can simply skip two to three meals and eat only when your plan says so. In other words, intermittent fasting ends your slavery to food.

- As you have to arrange for one or two meals each day, intermittent fasting reduces your grocery bill to 50%. This is beneficial for people who have difficulty arranging six meals per day. Moreover, it also saves time and energy.

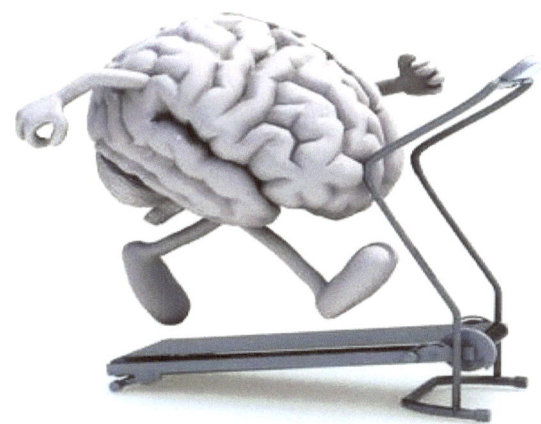

- A major misconception which some people in our society have is that fasting is harmful for brain health and that you should eat a banana every two hours or so. This misconception is based on the assumption that the brain needs a continuous intake of carbs for its proper functioning. But this concept has now been proved wrong. Scientists now believe that during fasting, B-hydroxybutyrate and acetoacetate replaces glucose, thus providing energy for brain metabolism (Brain Metabolism during Fasting, The Journal Of Clinical Investigation Vol. 46, 1967). Intermittent fasting also increases the production of BDNF, a hormone present in the brain which enhances the resistance of neurons from degeneration. Moreover, it also preserves memory and helps in the repairing of damaged nerve cells.

- Since the levels of insulin are lowered during fasting, the body uses the stored fats for the production of energy. As long as insulin levels are high in the body, the fats can't be burned as insulin is highly anabolic (taking chemical energy from food and transforming it into fats). This greatly helps in weight loss.

- The levels of the Human Growth Hormone (HGH) also become high during the fasting period. HGH helps in repairing of the body tissues and building muscles.

- During fasting, a process known as autophagy initiates in which the damaged and worn out cells of the body are repaired and recycled. Moreover, due to this process, the cells also get rid of waste materials.

- How often have you heard people saying that exercising with an empty stomach is harmful for health? But it is just another misconception. The truth is that exercising with an empty stomach is more beneficial than exercising with a full stomach. The reason behind this is that during starvation glycogen break down stops and the breakdown of fats starts.

This eventually results in a better metabolic activity, greater loss of fats and faster recovery from injuries.

Chapter 4: Cons of intermittent Fasting

In the previous chapter, the benefits of intermittent fasting were discussed. This chapter will discuss some of the demerits of intermittent fasting.

Some of the demerits of intermittent fasting are briefly discussed below:

- When a person is in the first week of this diet plan, he will feel weakness in his body. Moreover, he will also feel out of focus and hunger most of the times. The reason behind this isn't that your body isn't getting enough nutrients. The reason is that you have changed your dieting plan which you used to follow since you were very young. If you tolerate the first week, your body will adapt itself to this new change.

- A person has to face eating problems in intermittent fasting. He won't be able to follow the exact eating pattern after 16 hours of fasting. If you don't agree with me, picture yourself in the situation. You have just fasted for almost 16 hours. Now you will either eat too much or too little, both of which are harmful for the body. If you eat too much, you won't be able to reap out the benefits of this plan. On the other hand if you eat too little, you won't be able to perform your daily life activities during the fasting period. So intermittent fasting has to be adopted in its full essence as it isn't just about staying hungry; it is also about providing the body with the adequate amount of nutrients.

- Intermittent fasting might not be a good choice for people who are underweight. The reason is that its main focus is on cutting the unwanted fats from the body. Moreover, people having issues with their blood sugar levels and those suffering from hypoglycemia (abnormally low level of glucose in the blood) should avoid this plan.

Intermittent fasting has its own merit and demerits. But, unlike other dieting plans, it doesn't have any life threatening demerits. So, to see the true colors of intermittent fasting, you'll just have to bear with it for a week or two. It'll help you live a longer and happier life in the long run. So you should definitely give it a go.

Now that you know the merits and demerits of intermittent fasting, you might be wondering where the plan is. The wait is over! You just have to flip the page over as the next chapter will inform you about the different plans of intermittent fasting.

Chapter 5: How to Employ It In Your Daily Life

There are three major types of intermittent fasting. In each of the types, the fasting and the non-fasting schedules are different. The types are mentioned below:

Daily Fasting:

In this method of fasting, a person fasts for 16 hour and has the liberty of eating during the remaining 8 hours. This method is quite beneficial for overweight and obese people. One thing is important to mention that the 16 hours fast is recommended for men; women can fast for 10-14 hours. Age isn't a restriction in this fasting method. However, people with eating disorders and pregnant women should abstain from this method of fasting. The schedule for this fasting method is given in the following schedule:

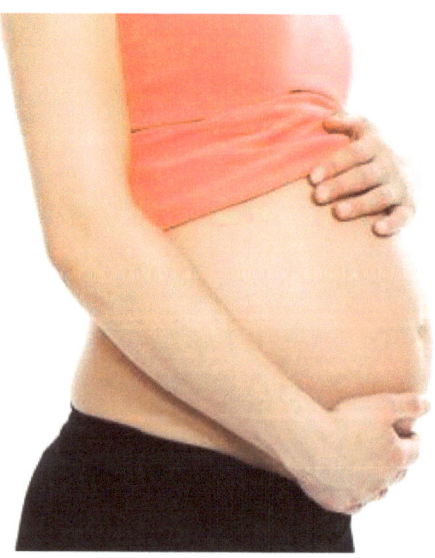

Sunday - Saturday (same schedule all week):

SLEEPING (Fasting) 8pm - 8 am
EATING 8 am - Noon & 4 pm - 8 pm
FASTING Noon - 4pm

Weekly Fasting:

This method of fasting is relatively easier as compared to daily fasting as an individual has to skip two meals only. In other words, you will have to fast on only one specific day of the week. This eating schedule is beneficial in the sense that you can eat every day of the week while still getting the benefits of a 24 hours fast. However, a person loses less weight as compared to daily fasting. The schedule of this fasting method is mentioned below:

Sunday - Saturday:
SLEEPING (Fasting) 8 pm - 8 am

* Now pick one 24 hour peroid out of the week (I suggest Monday to Tuesday) to fast from Noon until the next day at Noon.

Alternate Fasting:

As the name suggests, in this method the person fasts on alternate days of the week. For example if you eat on Monday night, then you will have to fast on Tuesday evening; you can eat again on Wednesday and fast on Thursday. This method is more beneficial than daily fasting in the sense that it gives longer time in the fasted state. Thus more benefits can be revived from this fasting method as compared to the previous mentioned fasting methods. The following table further clarifies the daily schedule for this fasting method:

Sunday - Saturday:
SLEEPING (Fasting): 8 pm - 8 am

* Alternating days fast from 4 pm - 4 pm the following day, then eat from 4 pm - 4 pm the following day.

Example: Monday start fasting at 4pm, start eating again on Tuesday at 4 pm, resume fasting Wednesday at 4pm, start eating at 4 pm Thursday, resume fast Friday at 4 pm, and this continues....

Chapter 6: How to Maximize the Benefits of Intermittent Fasting

Now that you have an idea about the types of intermittent fasting, we move towards the ways to reap out the maximum benefits from intermittent fasting. The following are some of the ways to obtain maximum benefits from intermittent fasting:

- You can celebrate a CHEAT DAY when you have fasted for a specific number of days which is dependent upon the fat present in the body. People who have 10% body fat can have cheat day after every 5 days; those with 14% body fat can cheat after every 9 days; those with 18% body fats can cheat once in every two week; those with 28% or more body fat can cheat once every month. The method of the diet is as simple as it sounds. On a specific cheat day you can eat whatever you want, whenever you want. There is no need to follow the schedules given by many other diet books about what to eat on a cheat day. Simply do whatever you want on the cheat day. It won't affect your past progress; it will enhance it.

- The main essence of intermittent fasting is to reduce the caloric intake. Therefore, your vitamin and nutrient intake shouldn't suffer as a result of intermittent fasting. If you feel that you aren't taking enough fruits and vegetables during the non-fasting period, you should go for the vitamin supplements. These supplements will fulfill your vitamin needs

- You have to follow the intermittent dieting plan in its full essence if you want to get the most out of it. Whichever type of intermittent fasting suits you best, follow it with all your heart and soul. Don't add foods on your own considering them as minor additions because these minor additions might prove harmful for you in the long run.

- Combining intermittent fasting with moderate exercise is a very good idea. Although exercising during starvation is beneficial, it's best that you exercise during the non-fasting period to avoid dizziness due to the low blood sugar level. You can adjust the intensity of exercise according to your fitness level. However, you should take plenty of water and supplements during the exercises.

- Taking green tea is quite beneficial as it has anti-oxidants and theanine in it; these two speeds up your rate of metabolism and protect the tissues from toxic material. Moreover, the low amount of caffeine promotes fat loss.

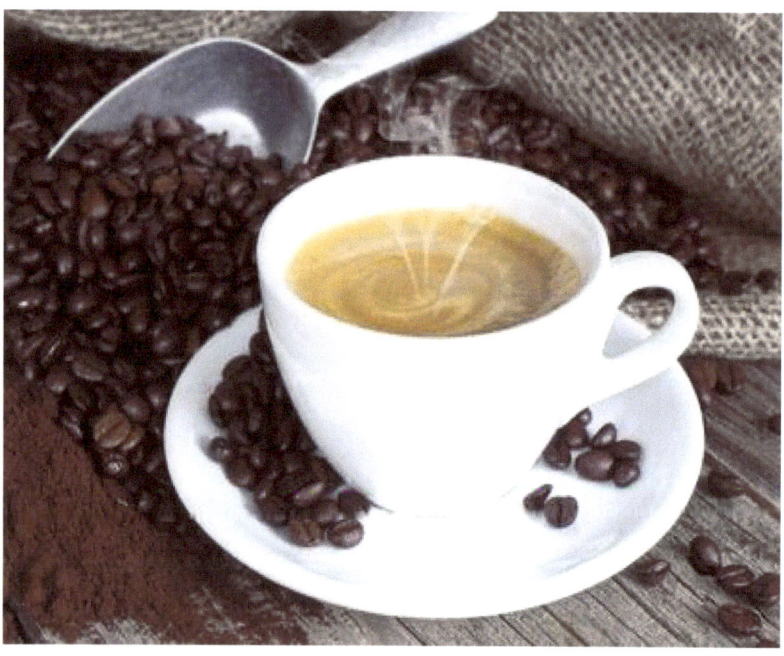

Section 3: Intermittent fating- A Boon for Health

Chapter 7: Loose Some Extra Pounds

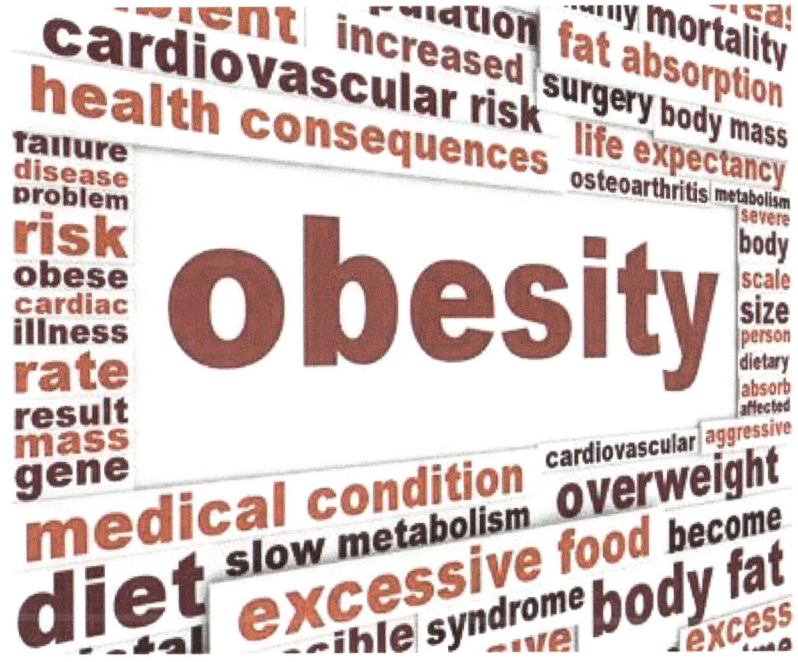

If you want to lose some extra pounds from your body, then you need to follow the intermittent fasting diet plan. Now you might be wondering that this statement is a bit of over exaggeration. But it isn't. This chapter will tell you all about how intermittent fasting helps in the weight loss process.

Now lets see whether the above mentioned statement is true or is it an over exaggeration. The main source of energy in our body is glucose. When a person eats, glucose is released into the blood stream. This leads to increase in the level of blood sugar levels in the body, which leads to an increase in the blood sugar levels in the body which releases a hormone known as insulin, the main role of which is the removal of extra sugar from the body, by stocking the sugar in the liver in the form of glycogen. But during eating the insulin levels become high. Hence, the conversion of fats to energy stops and the conversion of glucose to fats start. The main goal of fasting is to decrease this high level of insulin.

Now let's look at what happens during fasting. During fasting, the glycogen reserves are used up which lowers the blood sugar level in the body. This in turn lowers the insulin levels in the body. A hormone known as hormone sensitive leptin (HSL) is released during fasting. This hormone is beneficial for the body in the sense that it uses the calories from the stored body fats. Different studies have shown that fasting increases the production of the human growth hormone. Another hormone known as human growth hormone (HGH) is also released during fasting which burns fats.

So there you've it. The science behind how intermittent fasting helps in the fast loss process. But this is not all. You can maximize the weight loss effects of intermittent fasting by combining it with a healthy diet that is low in simple carbs and saturated fats and rich in complex carbs, proteins and unsaturated fats. Take one step further and combine your intermittent fasting and diet schedule with simple exercising plans like simple cardio, jogging and light body weight training exercises. So, what are you waiting for? Don't let the expensive weight loss dieting plans fool you anymore. Why spend thousands of dollars on useless dieting plans when you can try an amazing weight loss method at home- A method which is extremely cost effective, simple to follow and without any side effects.

Chapter # 8: Maximize your brain potential

The benefits of intermittent fasting on brain health are endless. These benefits range from improve in cognitive functions to cure of serious illnesses, cure of depression to improvement of brain neurotransmitter status. Its astounding that how something as simple as intermittent fasting can accomplish such wonders. But how so? Read the following text to know the reasons.

Fasting promotes brain cell autophagy.

In the previous chapters I discussed the concept of autophay. Let me repeat it to you again. Autophagy or self eating is a process in which cells get rid of their old and worn out parts. It's like a recycling process in which old components are recycled into new components. The benefits are quite self explanatory. How can a machine function properly if it is chocked with debris and wastes? Same is with human brain. Simply put, fasting is a way to renew the worn out brain neurons.

The validity of this fact was proved by a research done by The Scripps research institute, USA. According to the research, intermittent fasting and restriction of food intake induced profound autophay in brain neurons.

Fating boosts BDNF:

Intermittent fasting is the best way to boost the level of a key brain protein known as brain derived neurotropic factor or BDNF. But you might ask "What makes BDNF so important?" Several studies have proved the beneficial effects of BDNF on brain health. According to these researches, BDNF helps promote the development of new neurons- a process called "neurogenesis". It also has a neuroprotective role i.e. it protects existing neurons from damage. It also promotes the development of new synapses between neurons. Combining all these effects can significantly increase brain potentials like memory, cognition, learning and can even cure serious brain condition like Alzheimer's disease

Fating decreases the chances of stroke:

Who is not familiar with this word? There are several causes of stroke; the major reasons include cerebrovascular events, excessive release of inflammatory mediators, decrease of neuroprotective elements or due to some trauma. But the control to all this is within your reach. It's amazing that how something as simple as intermittent fasting can significantly reduce the risks of a lethal condition like stroke. Intermittent fasting accomplishes this wonder by increasing protection of neurons, increasing neuronal synapses and limiting neuronal breakdown by causing an increase in the release of BDNF- as described earlier. Moreover, fasting causes a significant decrease in the release of inflammatory mediators thus decreasing the chances of damage to brain blood vessels and cerebrovascular events- a leading cause of stroke.

Chapter # 9: Cure brain ailments.

Aging is an inevitable process and the effects of aging are seen in every organ. Human brain is affected in particular. The main problem starts when the rate of neuronal break down out paces the generation of new neurons. The result is serious brain complications like Alzheimer's disease, Huntington's disease and age related decline in learning and cognition. Intermittent fating is an effective cure for these conditions.

In addition, fasting finds its way as a solution to several psychiatric illnesses like depression, triggered by alteration in brain chemicals. Fasting normalizes the level of these chemicals and restores normal brain function. Read the coming text for detail.

Intermittent fasting for Alzheimer's cure:

All you need to know about the cause of Alzheimer's disease that it's caused due to the accumulation of degenerated brain proteins leading to characteristic features like decreased brain activity, poor cognition and poor learning. Research carried out by Institute on aging, USA proved the benefits of intermittent fasting on ameliorating the symptoms of Alzheimer's disease. The experiment was carried out on two groups of mice. One group followed dietary patterns similar to intermittent fasting and the other group didn't. The research proved that the first group showed a significant increase in brain potential as compared to the second group and showed a significant increase in learning and improved behaviour.

Intermittent fasting for Huntington's disease:

The most important cause of development and progression of Huntington's disease is poor glucose tolerance and decreased level of BDNF. A research carried out in John Hopkins's institute, USA showed the beneficial effects of intermittent fasting on mice that followed intermittent fating dietary model. These mice showed a significant increase in BDNF, neuroprotection, improved glucose tolerance, amelioration of symptoms of Huntington's disease and a significant decrease in the progression of this disease.

Intermittent fasting for Depression cure:

It's explained in the previous text that intermittent fasting causes a significant increase in the level of BDNF. Most of the anti-depressant medicines produce their therapeutic effects by causing an increase in the release of BDNF. So, the depression relieving effect of intermittent fasting is a well established fact now.

Chapter # 10: A cure for type II diabetes.

The first thing you need to know is that obesity is the major cause of type II diabetes. This is the type of diabetes in which the cells lose their responsiveness to Insulin. The cells get caught up into a net an excessive fat surrounding them and Insulin doesn't get a chance to find its way to the cells.

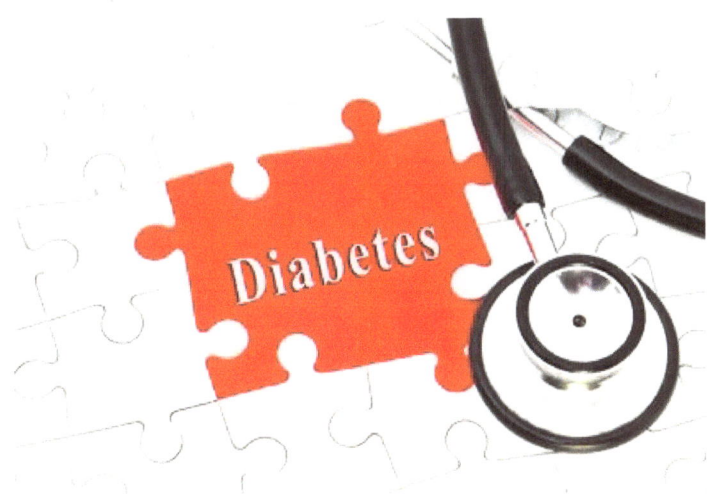

Type II diabetes can be cured by simple lifestyle changes that are focused on losing extra fat. Who has the time to go out and exercise? People find the solution to this problem by eating a handful of pills. It leads them nowhere and does more harm than good. If you don't have the time to exercise each day then intermittent fasting is the thing for you. Research has shown that intermittent fasting improves the level of glucose, sensitivity to insulin and slows the progression of symptoms in obese individuals with type II diabetes.

Another research proved that limiting the daily caloric intake to 600 calories per day can ameliorate the symptoms of type II diabetes. To eat so little is not possible for some individuals. So, it is better that you combine the principles of caloric restriction with those of intermittent fasting. The basic approach behind this technique is quite simple. Excessive calories are stored in the form of fats; you would remember that previous text. So, limited amount of calories when eaten at spaced intervals (intermittent fasting) can lead to a significant decrease in the level of fats and thus increase the sensitivity of cells to the effects of Insulin. The therapeutic efficacy of diabetes controlling drugs can also be increased when combined with intermittent fasting and planned eating schedule.

Chapter # 11: Strengthen your heart.

High blood pressure and heart attacks are prevalent in our societies like never before, thanks to the modern ways of living. All these problems arise when you make bad choices related to your way of living, especially unhealthy eating and minimal physical activity. Unhygienic eating and sedentary life style are forefront of thousands of ailments like obesity, type II diabetes and high level of cholesterol. All these factors, combined, result in a deadly outcome- heart attack. According to a research 80% of obese individuals that suffered from type II diabetes died of heart attack.

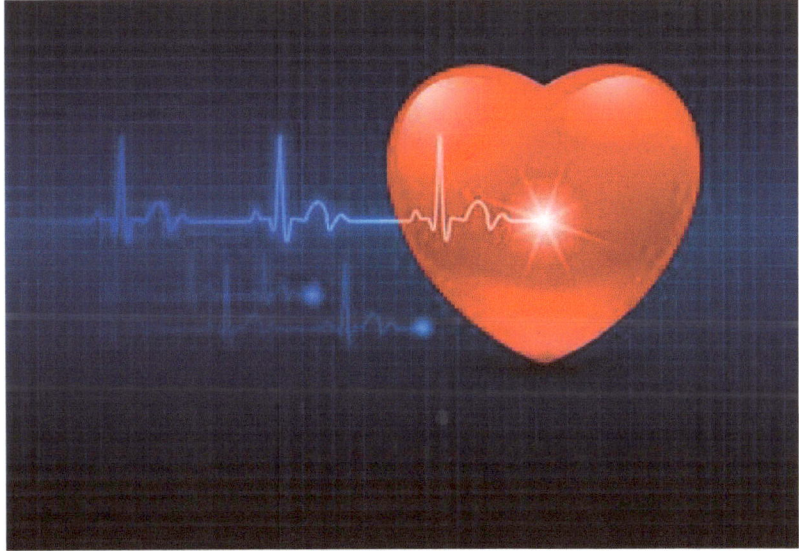

Intermittent fasting is an amazing therapeutic approach for those individuals that are facing a constant threat of heart attack and high blood pressure related complications. How great would it be if you could find a way to control your blood pressure and minimize the risks of heart attack with a natural way, which has got no side effect? Well, such solution is right within your reach. Intermittent fasting is what you're looking for. But at this point you might ask "How is fasting going to help me with my heart problem?" The answer is quite simple. You experience high blood pressure and risk of heart attack when your lipid profile is disturbed. A disturbed lipid profile is characterized by elevated level of bad fats and cholesterol. When these components exceed their normal limits, they start to occlude the lumen of blood vessels causing an increase in the level of blood pressure. The real problem arises when cholesterol occludes vessels supplying the heart. At fist partial occlusion may not develop some obvious symptoms but with passage of time this occlusion completely blocks these vessels and the result is heart attack. Intermittent fasting helps cure this condition by eliminating the root cause i.e. by lowering the level of bad fats and cholesterols. The result is healthy heart, controlled lipid profile and normal blood pressure.

The validity of this argument was proved by a study carried out at the University of Utah. The study concluded that 40% among 300 individuals those who fasted for at least once a day didn't develop occlusion of arteries. Moreover, following fasting regime for three weeks helps these individuals with controlling their level of cholesterol and bad fats.

Chapter # 12: Minimize oxidative stress.

Oxidative stress can be defined as an imbalance between body's potential to produce and detoxify damaging oxygen radicals. These reactive oxygen radicals can damage blood vessels and tissues resulting in a long of list of disorders. Some of these diseases are given below:

- Brain.
    - Bipolar disorder
    - Alzheimer
    - Anxiety
    - Parkinson
    - Stroke
- Vessels.
    - Atherosclerosis
    - Vasospasm
    - Hypertension
- Gastro-intestinal tract.
    - Pancreatitis'
    - Irritable bowel syndrome
    - Liver disease
- Lungs.
    - Acute respiratory distress syndrome
    - Asthma
- Multi-organ.
    - Chronic fatigue syndrome
    - Aging
    - Injury

- o Cancer
- Heart.
  - o Congestive heart failures
  - o Arrhythmia
  - o Angina
- Skin.
  - o Melanoma
  - o Dermatitis
  - o Psoriasis
- Joints.
  - o Osteoarthritis
  - o Arthritis
- Eyes.
  - o Cataractogenesis
  - o Retinal degeneration
  - o Macular degeneration
  - o Glaucoma
- Immune systems
  - o Autoimmune disorder
  - o Inflammation
  - o Allergies

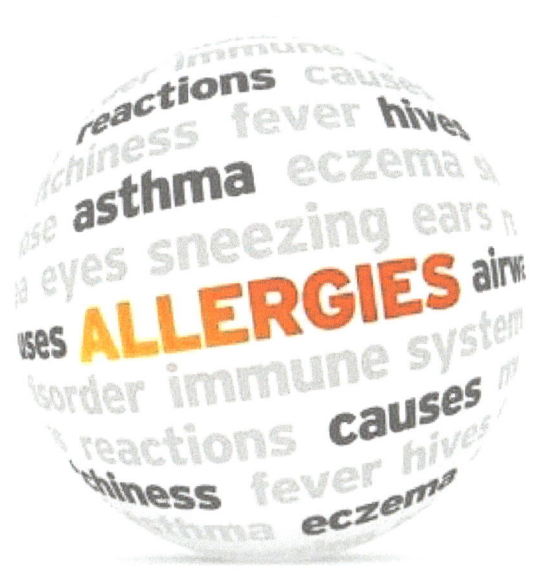

The above mentioned diseases are just a few among the long, never ending list of complications caused by oxidative stress. How fasting helps fight oxidative stress and diseases caused by it? Following mechanisms are most likely involved in reducing oxidative stress and its complications:

- First, fasting decreases the level of reactive oxygen species (ROS) - the real culprit behind oxidative damage.
- It breaks down old cell component through autophagy and decreases the production of reactive elements that would otherwise produced by their decomposition.
- It increases the production of certain chemicals that make cells resistant to oxidative damage e.g. BDNF reduces oxidative damage in brain tissues.

Section # 4: Conclusion. Intermittent Fasting – More Than A Diet Plan.

So in conclusion, intermittent fasting is more than a weigh loss method or ordinary diet plan. It's a complete life style. Not only does it provides a cure for obesity but also helps cure several other health complications related to heart, brain, lungs, kidney and joints. It's an amazing fact that how something as simple as intermittent fasting can do wonders. So what are you waiting for? Practice this way of living coupled with healthy diet and living style to reap the maximum benefits.

Photo credits:

female surgeon with surgical team

© *beerkoff - Fotolia.com*

human brain on a running machine

© *fabioberti.it - Fotolia.com*

Stressed

© *lassedesignen - Fotolia.com*

ÄrztinmitSchild - Diabetes

© *PhotographyByMK - Fotolia.com*

Allergies

© *kbuntu - Fotolia.com*

Diabetes

© *Marco2811 - Fotolia.com*

Diseased artery with fatty deposits

© *Giovanni Cancemi - Fotolia.com*

Obesity medical poster design

© *paradox - Fotolia.com*

Abstract Heart Monitor

© *dvarg - Fotolia.com*

Cholesterol plaque in artery (atherosclerosis) illustration

© *Diamond_Images - Fotolia.com*

Gothic valentine

© *grandeduc - Fotolia.com*

Beautiful pregnant belly

© *SergejsRahunoks - Fotolia.com*

Author Bio

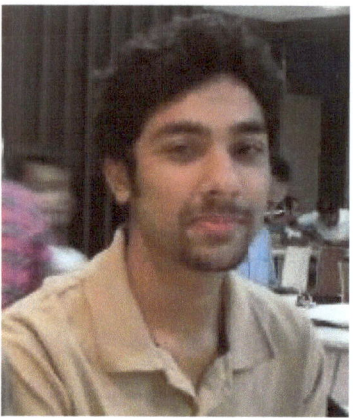

Muhammad Usman is a distinguished medical graduate of Allama iqbal medical college (AIMC). He is a professional writer who has been in the field for more than 4 years. During this time he has produced 10,000+ articles, blogs and eBooks on various niches related to diseases, health, fitness, nutrition and well being. He is a regular contributor to several journals related to medicine and surgery. He is the editor of several journals and newspapers.

Check out some of the other JD-Biz Publishing books
Gardening Series on Amazon

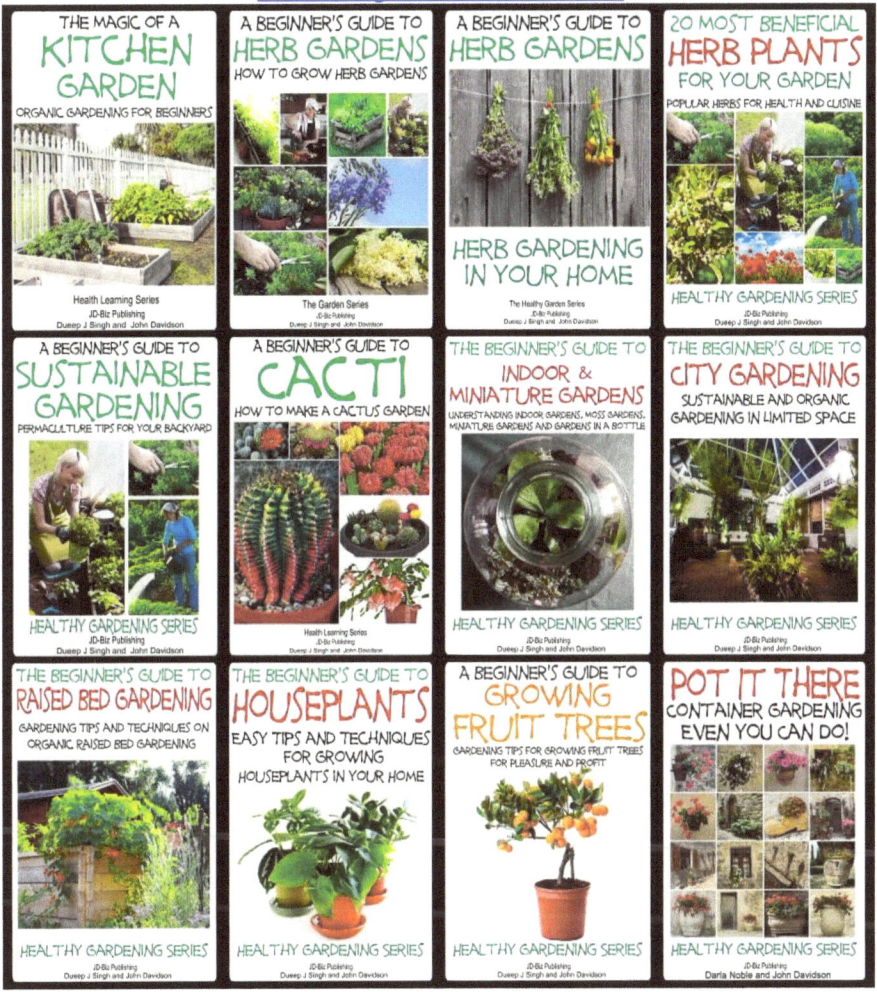

Download Free Books!
http://MendonCottageBooks.com

Health Learning Series

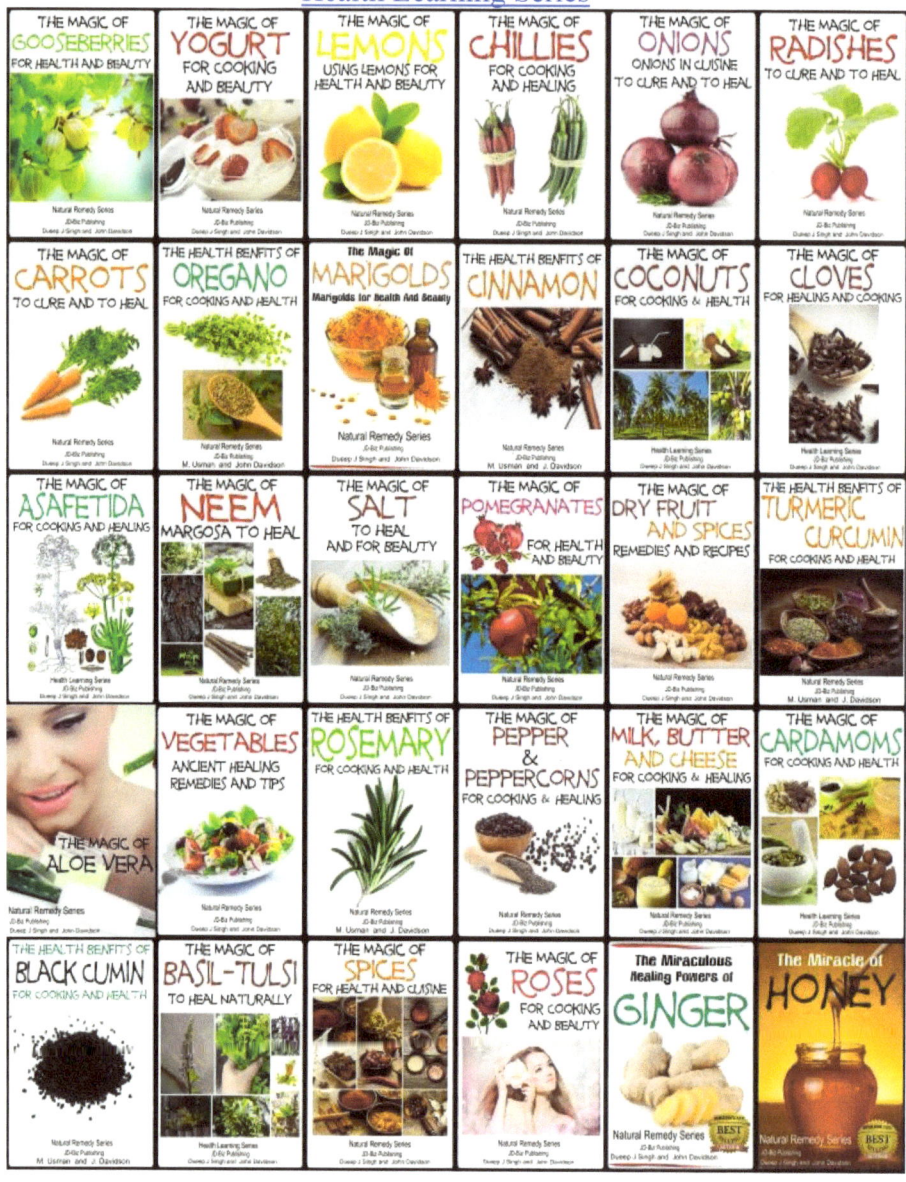

Country Life Books

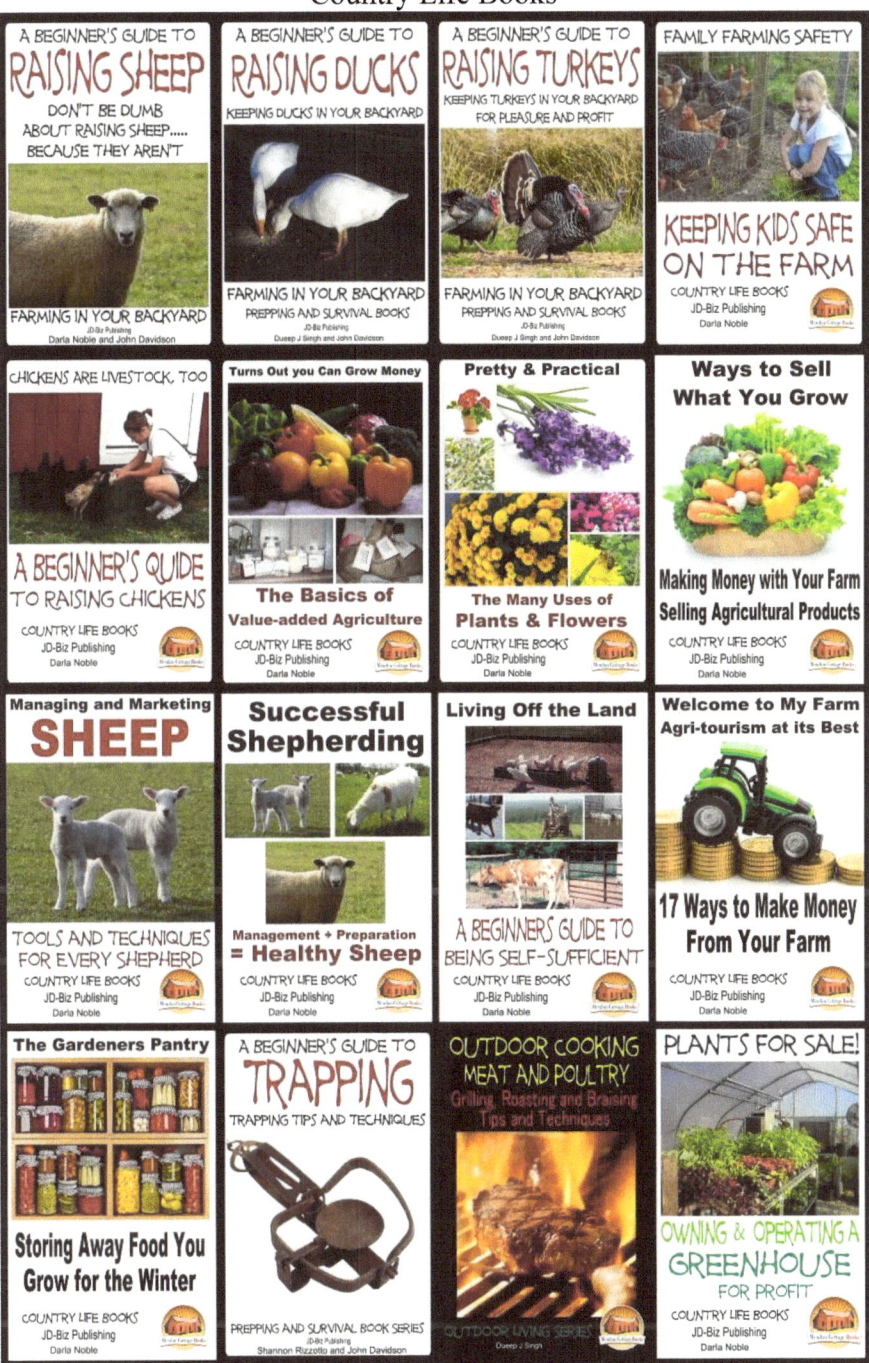

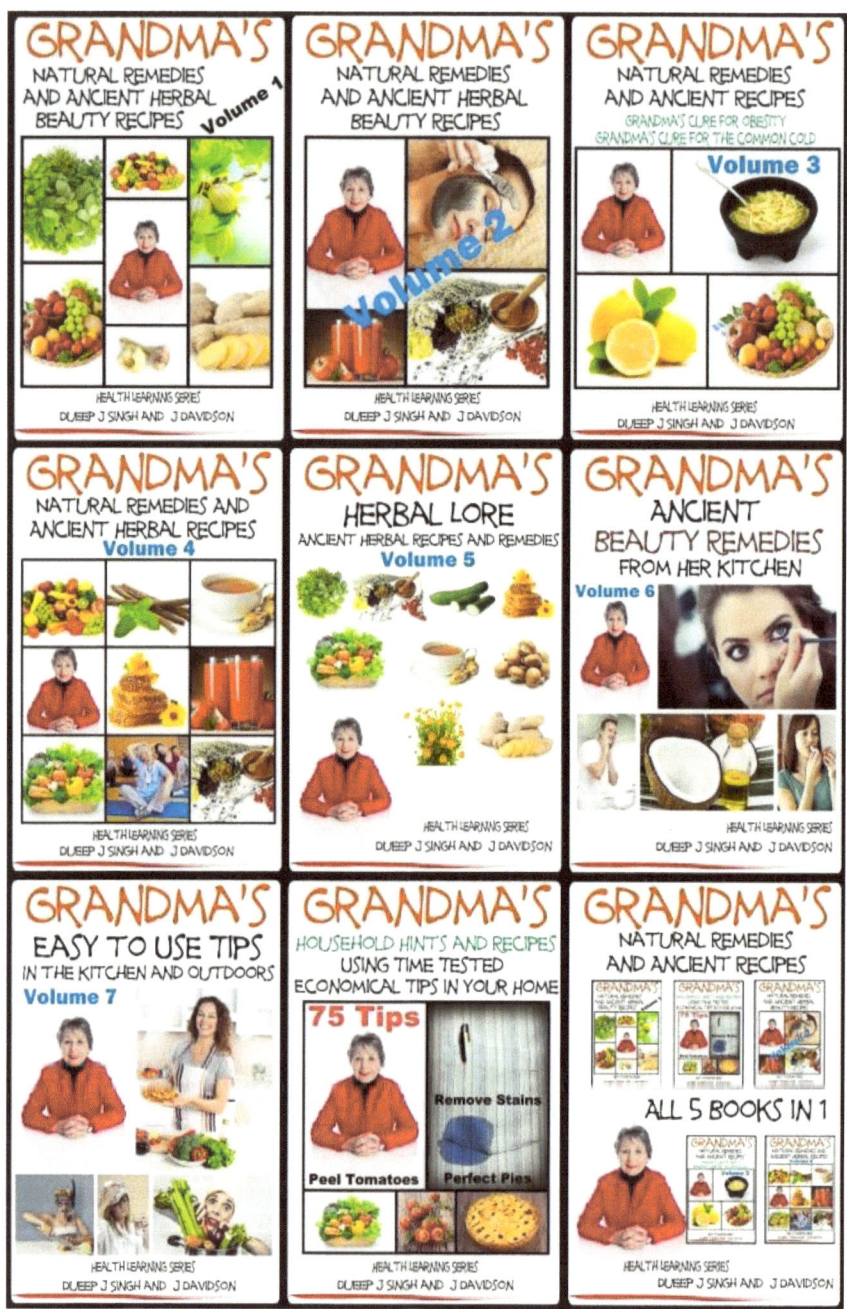

Health Learning Series

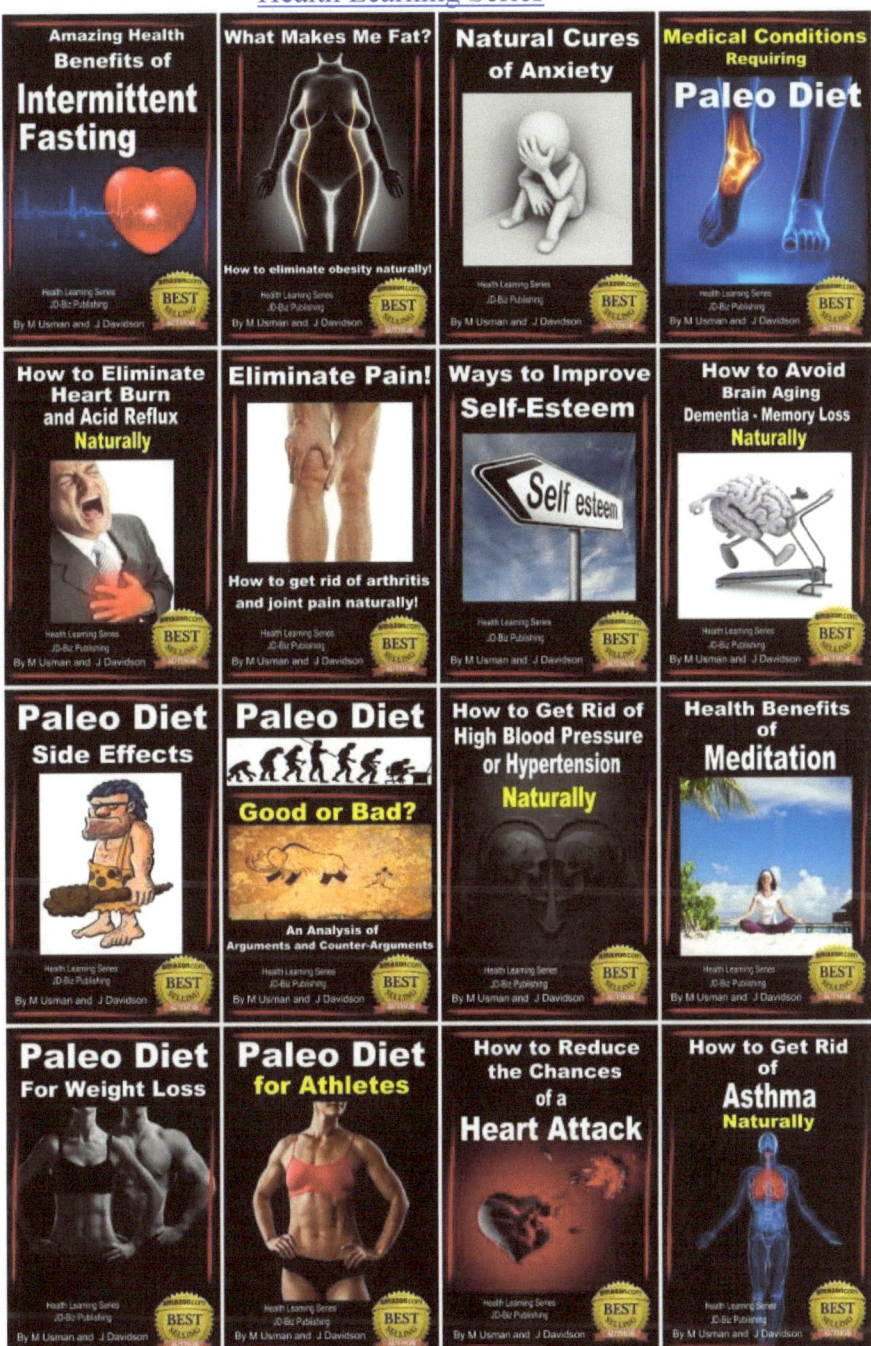

Amazing Animal Book Series

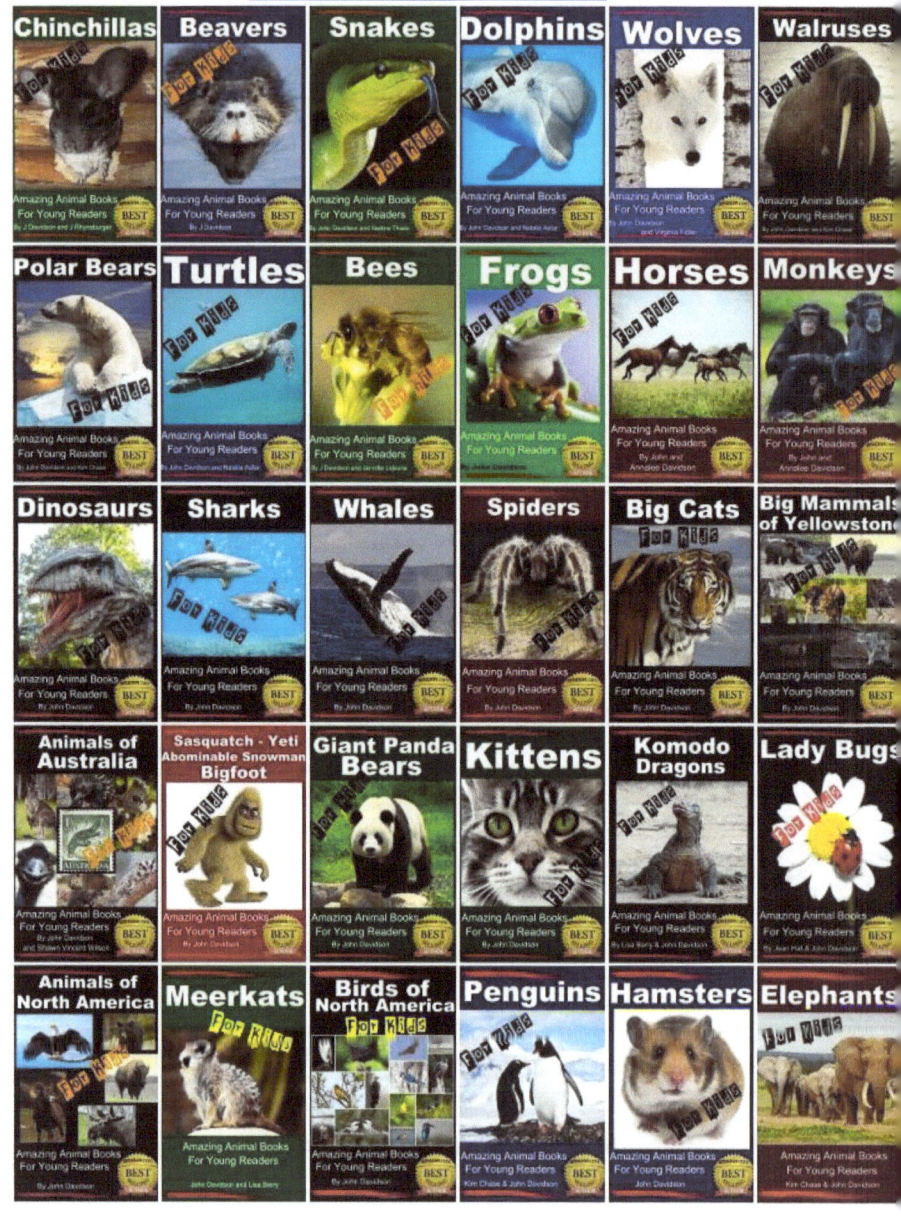

Learn To Draw Series

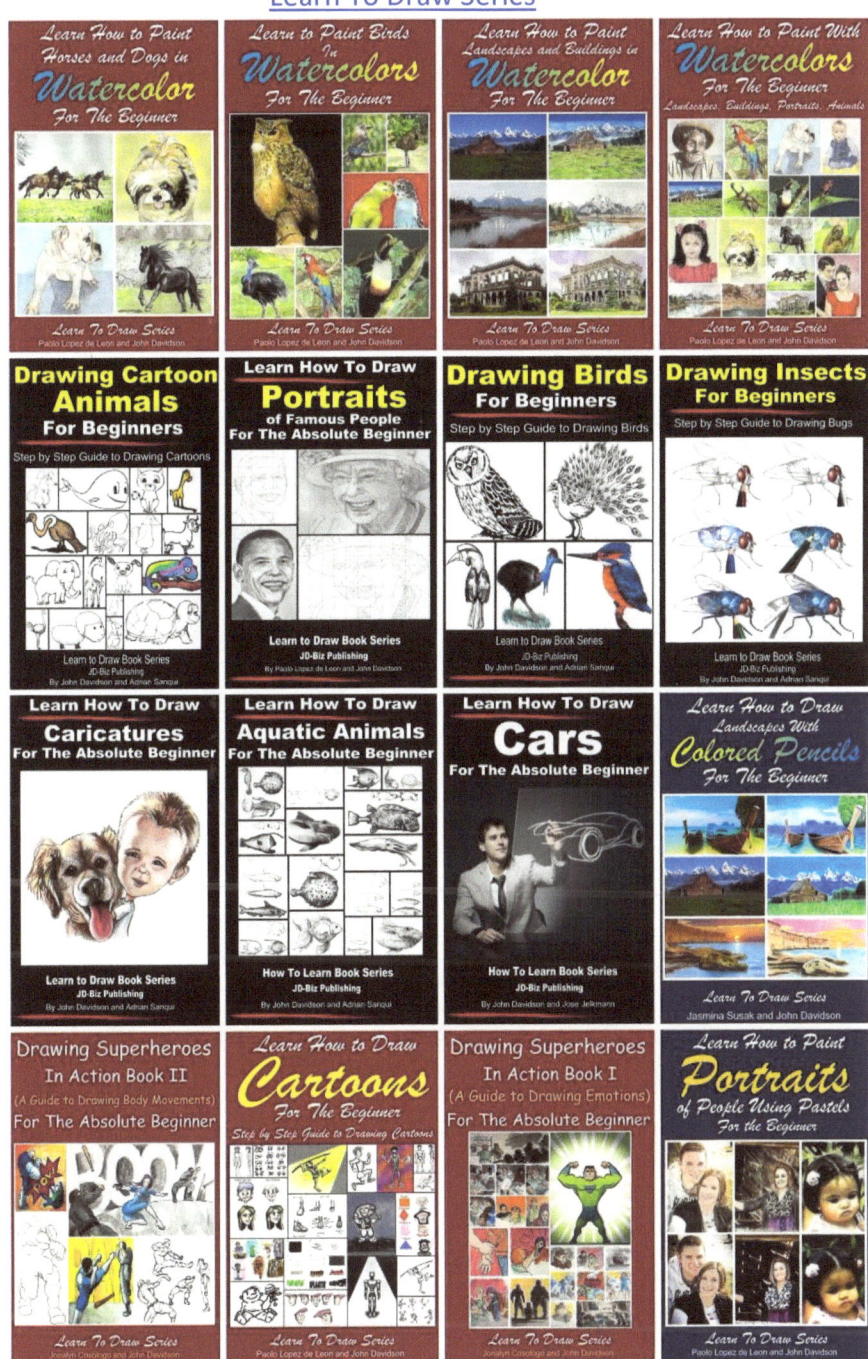

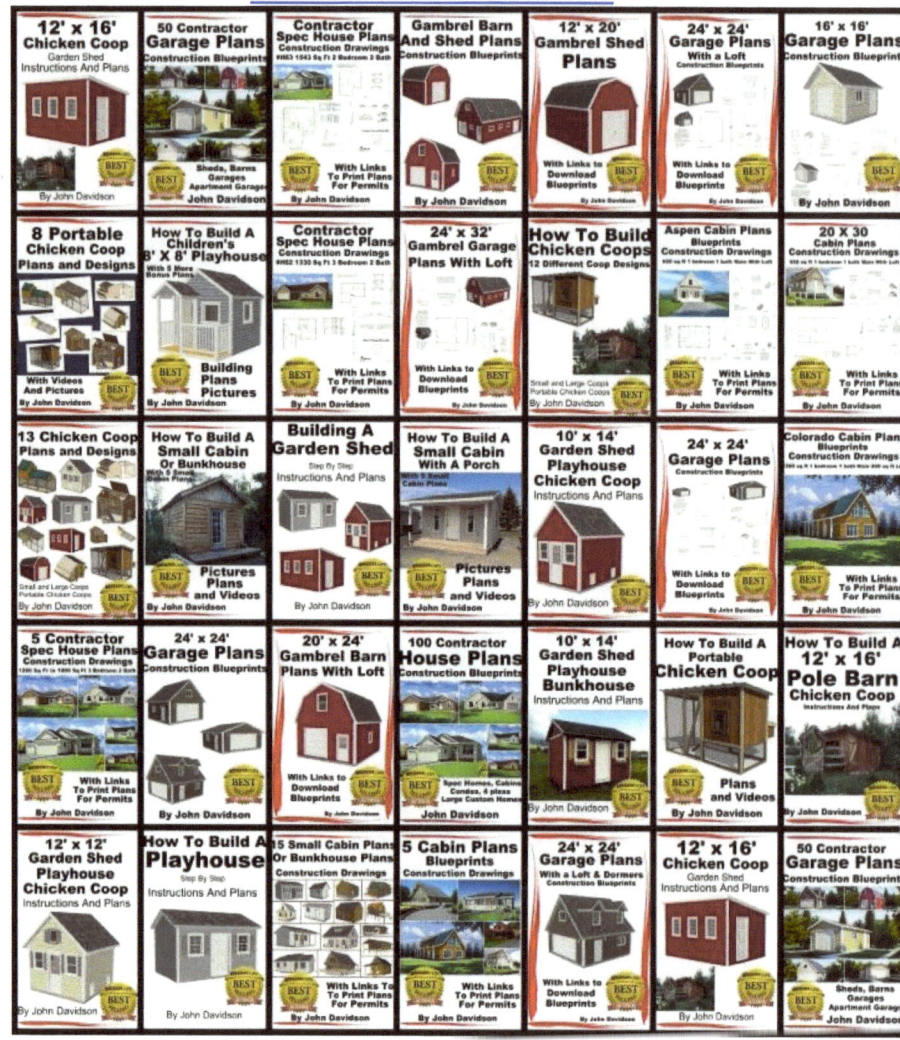

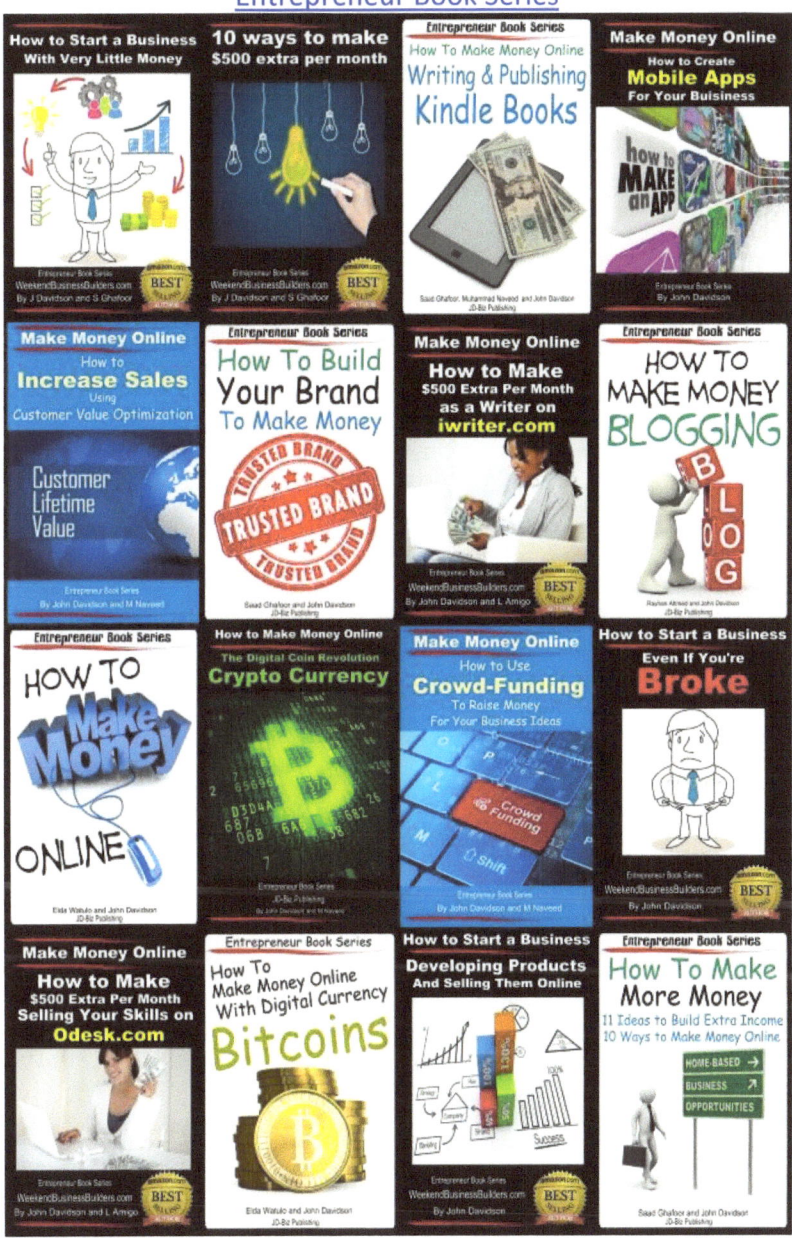

Our books are available at

1. Amazon.com
2. Barnes and Noble
3. Itunes
4. Kobo
5. Smashwords
6. Google Play Books

Download Free Books!
http://MendonCottageBooks.com

Publisher

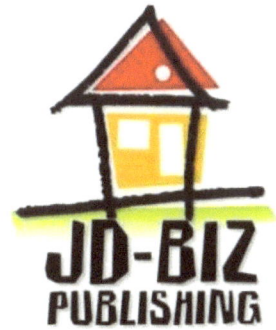

JD-Biz Corp

P O Box 374

Mendon, Utah 84325

http://www.jd-biz.com/

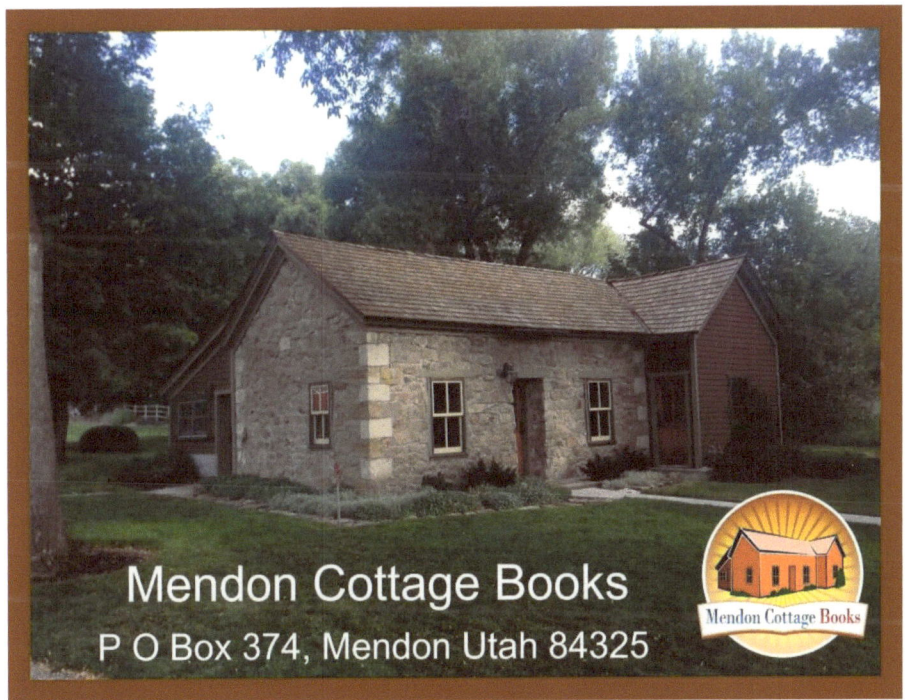

www.ingramcontent.com/pod-product-compliance
Lightning Source LLC
Chambersburg PA
CBHW050835290526
45792CB00001B/397

* 9 7 8 1 5 1 7 6 6 1 7 2 4 *